I0830988

Table of Contents

Melanoma, the most serious type of skin cancer, develops in the cells (melanocytes) that produce melanin — the pigment that gives your skin its color. Melanoma can also form in your eyes and, rarely, inside your body, such as in your nose or throat.

The exact cause of all melanomas isn't clear, but exposure to ultraviolet (UV) radiation from sunlight or tanning lamps and beds increases your risk of developing melanoma. Limiting your exposure to UV radiation can help reduce your risk of melanoma.

The risk of melanoma seems to be increasing in people under 40, especially women. Knowing the warning signs of skin cancer can help ensure that cancerous changes are detected and treated before the cancer has spread. Melanoma can be treated successfully if it is detected early.

MELANOMA DIET RECIPES

BREAKFAST

1.Apple Cranberry Bread Pudding

Prep Time: 20 mins

Cook Time: 50 mins

Total Time: 70 mins

Yield: 12 Servings

Ingredients

- 4 large eggs
- ½ cup brown sugar, divided
- 4 cups milk
- 2 teaspoons pure vanilla extract
- 1 loaf brioche or sourdough bread, cubed
- 2 ½ tablespoons butter, divided
- 2 medium firm apples, diced
- 1 cup cranberries
- ½ orange, juiced
- 1 ½ teaspoons ground cinnamon

- ¼ teaspoon ground nutmeg
- 1 cup Quaker granola
- Maple syrup, for serving

Instructions

1. In a mixing bowl whisk together eggs and ¼ cup brown sugar. Whisk in milk and vanilla extract.

2. Place cubed bread in a greased 9×13 glass or ceramic baking dish. Pour milk mixture over the bread and stir to combine. Allow to sit 15-20 minutes. Preheat the oven to 350 degrees.

3. In a large saucepan, melt 2 tablespoons butter. Add apples, cranberries, remaining ¼ cup brown sugar and orange juice; stir to combine. Bring to a simmer and allow to cook 4-5 minutes, until fruit just starts to soften. Stir in cinnamon and nutmeg.

4. Pour apple/cranberry mixture over the bread mixture and stir to combine. Bake 40 minutes.

5. In a small glass mixing bowl, melt remaining ½ tablespoon butter. Stir in granola to combine. Top bread mixture with granola mixture. Bake an

additional 10-20 minutes, until top is puffed and light golden brown. Allow to slightly cool and serve with maple syrup.

2. Cheesy Wonton Breakfast Cups

Prep Time: 10 mins

Cook Time: 25 mins

Total Time: 35 mins

Yield: 12 Breakfast Cups

Ingredients

- 12 wonton wrappers
- 1 cup spinach, chopped
- 1 link smoked spicy chicken sausage, chopped
- ¼–½ cup shredded sharp cheddar cheese
- 12 large eggs
- Pinch coarse salt and ground black pepper
- Pinch crushed red pepper flakes (optional)
- 1 scallion, sliced

Instructions

1. Preheat oven to 350 degrees.

2. Grease a 12-cup muffin tin. Tuck wonton wrappers into each muffin cup. Coat with cooking spray or brush with oil/butter. Bake 5-6 minutes, until just starting to brown. Remove from the oven.

3. Distribute spinach, sausage, cheese and an egg in each wonton cup. Season each with salt, black pepper and crushed red pepper flakes.

4. Bake 18-19 minutes, until egg is just set. Garnish with sliced scallions.

3. Loaded Breakfast Tostadas

Prep Time: 10 mins

Cook Time: 10 mins

Total Time: 20 mins

Yield: 8 Tostadas

Ingredients

Beans:

- 1 (15-ounce) can black beans, drained and rinsed
- 1 (4.5-ounce) can diced green chilies
- 2 tablespoons water
- ½ teaspoon ground cumin
- Coarse salt and ground black pepper

Tostadas:

- 2 slices cooked bacon, crumbled
- 8 large eggs
- Coarse salt and ground black pepper
- 8 tostada shells*
- 2 ripe avocados, sliced

- ½ cup salsa

- ¼ cup fresh cilantro, chopped

Instructions

1. Heat oven to a low broil.

2. In a medium saucepan, heat black beans, green chilies, water, cumin and a pinch of salt and black pepper to medium heat. Bring to a simmer, stirring regularly. Use the back of a fork to smash some of the beans.

3. Heat large non-stick skillet to medium. Add bacon and cook until crispy, about 3-4 minutes on each side. Remove and place on a paper towel. Once slightly cooled, crumble. Discard most of the bacon fat. Place the skillet back on medium heat. Add eggs and season with salt and pepper. Allow to cook 2-3 minutes, until white is mostly cooked. Place a lid on top and cook an additional 1-2 minutes, until white is completely cooked but yolk is runny. Remove from heat.

4. Place tostadas under the broiler and allow to cook 1-2 minutes on each side.

5. Spread beans on the tostadas, then top with eggs, crumbled bacon, avocado, salsa and cilantro.

4. Spiced Pumpkin Bread

Prep Time: 5 mins

Cook Time: 55 mins

Total Time: 60 mins

Yield: 1 loaf (~12 slices)

Ingredients

- 1 (15-ounces) can pumpkin puree
- 3 tablespoons oil
- 3 large eggs
- ½ cup brown sugar
- 1 cup oat flour (or whole wheat pastry, whole wheat, all-purpose)
- 1 ½ teaspoons baking powder
- ¾ teaspoon baking soda
- ¾ teaspoon coarse salt
- ¾ teaspoon ground cinnamon
- ¼ teaspoon ground nutmeg
- ¼ teaspoon ground ginger
- Pinch ground cloves
- 1 tablespoon granulated sugar

Instructions

1. Preheat oven to 350 degrees.

2. In a medium bowl, whisk together pumpkin puree, oil, eggs and brown sugar until combined.

3. In a separate medium bowl, whisk together flour, baking powder, baking soda, salt, cinnamon, nutmeg, ginger and cloves. Add dry ingredients to wet ingredients, slowly, whisking until just combined.

4. Pour batter into a greased loaf pan. Sprinkle top with granulated sugar. Bake 55-65 minutes, until toothpick inserted in center comes out almost clean.

5. Crispy Hash Brown Haystacks

Prep Time: 5-10 mins

Cook Time: 15-20 mins

Total Time: 20-30 mins

Yield: Serves 6

Ingredients

Hash Brown Haystacks:

- 3 cups frozen hash brown potatoes
- 6 large eggs
- ¼ cup sour cream or plain Greek yogurt
- 1 ½ tablespoons fresh dill, chopped
- 1 tablespoon fresh chives, chopped
- ¾ teaspoon garlic powder
- ¾ teaspoon coarse salt
- ½ teaspoon onion powder
- ¼ teaspoon ground black pepper
- 2 tablespoons oil

Fried Eggs:

- 6 large eggs

- Coarse salt and ground black pepper

- Green onion and sour cream or plain Greek yogurt, for serving

Instructions

1. Place hash browns, eggs, sour cream/Greek yogurt, dill, chives, garlic powder, salt, onion powder and black pepper in a large bowl. Mix until completely combined. Heat oil in a large nonstick or cast iron skillet. Place dollops of hash brown mixture into hot skillet. Allow to cook 2-3 minutes on each side, or until crispy on each side. Repeat with remaining mixture.

2. Coat a medium frying pan with cooking spray and heat to medium. Crack eggs into the pan once it's hot and season with salt and black pepper. Allow to cook for a few seconds, then turn heat down to medium-low. Allow to cook until egg white is almost set, then put a lid on the pan and turn to low. Cook just until top of the white is set, but yolk is completely uncooked.

3. Place eggs on crispy hash brown haystacks and serve
    with green onion or sour cream/Greek yogurt.

6. Healthy Morning Glory Muffins

Prep Time: 10-15 mins

Cook Time: 18-22 mins

Total Time: 28-37 mins

Yield: 12 muffins

Ingredients

- 2 cups old-fashioned oats
- ¼ cup almond meal
- 2 tablespoons ground flax seed
- 2 teaspoons baking soda
- 2 teaspoons cinnamon
- 1 teaspoon ground ginger
- 1 teaspoon ground nutmeg
- ¾ teaspoon coarse salt
- 3 large eggs
- ½ cup dark brown sugar
- 1 cup plain or vanilla Greek yogurt
- 2 teaspoon vanilla extract
- 2 tablespoon oil
- 2 cups carrots, finely shredded

- 1 medium granny smith apple, skin on, finely shredded
- ½ cup raisins
- ½ cup shredded or grated unsweetened coconut
- ½ cup chopped walnuts

Instructions

1. Preheat oven to 375 degrees. Prepare 12-cup muffin tin with muffin tin liners coated with cooking spray.

2. In the bowl of a stand mixer and using the paddle attachment, combine oats, almond meal, flax seed, baking soda, cinnamon, ginger, nutmeg and salt.

3. In a separate mixing bowl, whisk together eggs, brown sugar, yogurt, vanilla extract and canola oil. Fold in carrots, apple, raisins and ¼ cup coconut.

4. Turn the stand mixer on low and slowly add the wet ingredients to the dry. Mix until just combined (do not over mix).

5. Scoop a heaping ¼ cup of muffin mix into each liner. Top each with remaining coconut and chopped

walnuts. Bake for 18-22 minutes, until toothpick inserted into the center comes out clean. Allow to cool on a wire rack.

7. Walnut Chai Pancakes

Prep Time: 5-10 mins

Cook Time: 10-15 mins

Total Time: 15-25 mins

Yield: 6 pancakes

Ingredients

- 1 ½ cups whole wheat pastry flour
- 4 teaspoons chai tea leaves (out of 4 tea bags)
- 2 teaspoons baking powder
- ¼ teaspoon coarse salt
- 1 ¼ cups low fat buttermilk
- 2 large eggs
- 2 tablespoons oil
- 2 tablespoons brown sugar
- 1 ½ tablespoon vanilla extract
- ½ cup vanilla yogurt
- ½ cup chopped walnuts

Instructions

1. In the bowl of a stand mixer, combine flour, chai tea leaves, baking powder and salt.

2. In a separate bowl, whisk together buttermilk, eggs, canola oil, brown sugar and vanilla extract.

3. Turn mixer on medium speed and slowly pour wet ingredients into the dry and allow to whisk until batter is smooth.

4. Heat a saute pan or cast iron skillet to medium-high heat and coat with cooking spray. Pour about ¼ cup batter into the pan. Cook until bubbles start to form on the top; flip and cook another 30-60 seconds, until bottom has browned.

5. Stack pancakes and top with vanilla yogurt and walnuts.

Prep Time: 10 minutes

Cook Time: 10 minutes

Servings: 4

Ingredients

- 1 15-ounce can black beans rinsed
- 1 cup jarred salsa made from red or green chiles (or a mix), mild, medium or hot
- 1 cup nut milk unsweetened and unflavored (such as almond, cashew, macadamia, pecan, or other)
- ½ teaspoon kosher salt
- 4 to 6 large eggs
- 1 avocado sliced
- 1 scallion both white and green parts finely chopped (optional)
- Corn tortillas warmed

Instructions

1. Combine the beans, salsa, nut milk, and salt in a large skillet. Bring to a gentle simmer over medium heat. Use a spoon to make a well in the sauce and crack an egg into it. Repeat with as many eggs as you want to cook and that your skillet allows.

2. Cover tightly and adjust the heat so that the sauce is gently bubbling at a low simmer. Cook for 5 to 8 minutes, depending on how you like your eggs: about 7 minutes for a jammy yolk or longer for a fully cooked one.

3. To serve, scoop out some of the sauce and an egg or two into each bowl. Top with avocado slices and scatter with scallions, if using. Serve with warm tortillas on the side.

9. Pasta Cauliflower Alfredo

Prep Time: 25 minutes

Cook Time: 20 minutes

Servings: 6

Ingredients

- 1 head cauliflower medium-sized
- 1/2 teaspoon kosher or sea salt
- 1 cup raw cashews soaked for at least one hour and drained
- 1 teaspoon truffle salt
- 2 tablespoons nutritional yeast
- 1/4 tsp white pepper
- 1 pound whole grain pasta

Instructions

1. Trim the cauliflower of any discolored leaves. Trim the base of the main stem so that it stands upright. Place the whole head, stem side down, in a pan large

enough to contain it when covered. Add water to cover the stem and just the bottom of the cauliflower.

2. Place over high heat, bring to a boil and cover. Reduce the heat to low-medium. Steam for 15 minutes, or until the cauliflower is very soft and a knife or skewer easily pierces through to the core. Steaming times will vary depending on the size of your cauliflower — about 13 minutes for small, 15 minutes for medium, and 18 minutes for a large head.

3. Using tongs or a kitchen towel, transfer the cauliflower to a cutting board. Pour the cooking water into a measuring cup. Remove the leaves and cut them into slivers. Cut the stem from the rest of the head, trim off any woody parts, and chop into 2-inch pieces. Cut the head of cauliflower into 4 or 5 pieces.

4. Place the steamed cauliflower florets and pieces of stem in a blender. Add the cashews, truffle salt, nutritional yeast, white pepper and 3/4 cup of the cooking water. Blend on medium speed until combined, then on high speed until very creamy, about 2 minutes. Add more cooking water, if needed,

to create a pourable, smooth cauliflower cream. Set aside.

5. To cook the pasta, bring a large pot of water to a boil. Add 1 teaspoon of sea salt and add the pasta. Cook until al dente, or still chewy and not quite done. Drain over a colander.

6. Pour the cauliflower cream into the same pan used to cook the pasta. Warm over medium heat until bubbling gently. Add the cooked pasta to the sauce and gently combine with a wooden spoon. Once the pasta is coated with the alfredo sauce, add the slivered cauliflower leaves and warm through.

10. Zoodles with Almond Butter Sesame Sauce

Prep Time: 25 minutes

Servings: 4

Ingredients

- 2 medium zucchini
- 1/2 teaspoon sea salt
- 2 medium carrots
- 1 cucumber
- 1/2 cup smooth almond butter
- 1/4 cup extra virgin olive oil
- 1 tablespoon toasted sesame oil
- 1/4 cup low sodium soy sauce or gluten-free tamari
- 1/4 cup rice vinegar
- 1-2 tablespoons sambal oelek chili paste
- 1 tablespoon honey
- 1 teaspoon minced garlic
- 1 teaspoon grated or minced ginger
- 1 teaspoon grated fresh turmeric or 1/2 teaspoon dried
- black sesame seeds or toasted sesame seeds optional

- finely chopped scallion optional
- finely chopped red bell pepper optional

Instructions

1. Spiralize the zucchini using the "spaghetti" blade (ie the green blade of an OXO spiralizer, or the C blade of the Inspiralizer.) Place in a colander and toss with 1 teaspoon kosher or sea salt. Trim with scissors. Place the colander in the sink to drain while you make the rest of the recipe. (The salt will help draw out the water so the zucchini won't be soggy.)

2. Spiralize the carrots and the cucumber. Place in a large serving bowl.

3. To make the sauce, place the almond butter, extra virgin olive oil, sesame oil, soy sauce, rice vinegar, sambal oelek, honey, garlic, ginger, and turmeric in a blender or food processor and blend until smooth. Thin with small amounts of water, if necessary, to create a pourable sauce. Taste. Adjust for sweet, salty and spicy by adding more honey, soy sauce or sambal

oelek. If it needs to taste brighter, add a touch more
vinegar.

4. Prep any additional toppings, if using: diced red
    pepper, scallions, sesame seeds.

5. Just before serving, rinse the zoodles under cold water
    and shake dry in the colander. Transfer to a clean
    kitchen towel in a single layer and roll up to blot dry.
    Or, spin dry in a salad spinner. Place the zoodles in
    the serving bowl with the cucumber and carrot
    noodles.

6. Toss the noodles with the almond butter sesame
    sauce. Sprinkle with toppings, if using, and serve
    immediately.

11. Greek Salad with Feta Vinaigrette

Prep Time: 15 mins

Cook Time: 0 mins

Total Time: 15 mins

Yield: Serves 4

Ingredients

Feta Vinaigrette

- Zest and juice of 1 medium lemon (about ¼ cup)
- 2 tablespoons red wine vinegar
- 2 cloves garlic, peeled and minced
- 1 tablespoon granulated sugar + 1 tsp. honey
- 1 teaspoon dried oregano leaves
- ½ teaspoon dried basil leaves
- ½ cup extra virgin olive oil
- Dash coarse salt and ground black pepper
- ¼ cup crumbled feta cheese

Greek Salad

- 3 heads romaine lettuce, chopped

- 1 English cucumber, halved and thinly sliced

- 1 green bell pepper, thinly sliced

- ½ pint cherry tomatoes

- ½ cup pitted kalamata olives

- ½ cup crumbled feta cheese

- Dash coarse salt and ground black pepper

- ¼ cup shaved Parmesan cheese

- Whole pepperoncini, for garnish (optional)

Instructions

1. Whisk together lemon zest and juice, vinegar, garlic, sugar, honey, oregano and basil. Drizzle in olive oil until combined. Season with salt and black pepper and taste; adjust seasoning if necessary. Whisk in feta cheese. Set aside.

2. In a large bowl, combine romaine lettuce, cucumber, bell pepper, tomatoes, olives and feta cheese. Toss with desired amount of dressing. Sprinkle with coarse salt and black pepper and top with Parmesan cheese and garnish with pepperoncini, if desired.

12. Spinach, Strawberry & Fennel Salad

Prep Time: 15 min

Cook Time: 0 min

Total Time: 15 min

Yield: Serves 4

Ingredients

For the dressing:

- ½ cup plain yogurt (not Greek)
- 2 tablespoons mayonnaise
- 2 ½ tablespoons honey or granulated sugar
- 2 tablespoons apple cider vinegar
- 2 tablespoons fresh lemon zest and juice
- 1 tablespoon poppy seeds
- ¼ teaspoon kosher or sea salt

For the salad:

- 6 cups fresh spinach
- 2 cups fresh strawberries, hulled and sliced
- 2 medium avocados, sliced

- 1 small fennel bulb, thinly sliced

- ½ cup sugar snap peas, thinly sliced

- ¼ cup sliced almonds

Instructions

1. In a medium bowl, whisk together yogurt, mayonnaise, honey or sugar, apple cider vinegar, lemon zest and juice, poppy seeds and salt. Taste and adjust seasoning, if necessary.

2. Arrange spinach on 4 plates. Evenly distribute strawberries, avocado, fennel, snap peas and almonds. Drizzle with dressing just before serving.

Prep Time: 10 minutes

Cook Time: 15 minutes

Servings: 4

Ingredients

- 4 4-ounce pieces boneless, skin-on cod filets about 1-inch thick
- ½ cup fresh orange juice plus 2 tablespoons zest
- ⅓ cup fresh lemon juice plus 2 tablespoons zest
- 1 teaspoon kosher salt divided, plus more to taste
- 1 ¾ cups water
- 1 cup quinoa rinsed
- 1 medium zucchini spiralized, about 3 cups
- 3 tablespoons extra virgin olive oil plus more for coating the paper
- 2 medium garlic cloves thinly sliced
- ¼ teaspoon freshly ground black pepper
- 2 blood oranges very thinly sliced into half-moons
- Flaky salt to finish
- Cilantro leaves optional

Instructions

1. Preheat your oven to 400°F.

2. Place the cod in a 1-quart-size rimmed baking dish and pour the juices over them. Flip the fish over a few times so that the pieces are coated with the marinade, then place skin-side down. Sprinkle with ½ teaspoon of the salt, cover, and place in the fridge for at least 20 minutes and up to 1 hour.

3. While the cod marinates, cook the quinoa. Combine the water and quinoa in a medium saucepan with a tight-fitting lid and bring to a boil. Reduce the heat to a low simmer and cook for 15 minutes. Remove the pot from the heat, covered, and let it sit for 10 more minutes. Fluff with a fork when ready to use.

4. Meanwhile, place the zucchini in a medium bowl with the orange and lemon zests, oil, garlic, pepper, and the remaining ½ teaspoon salt. Toss well to coat and set aside.

5. To assemble the packets, lay out four 10-by-14-inch pieces of parchment paper. Fold each sheet in half, forming a 7-by-10-inch rectangle. Use scissors to cut

out a half-moon as big as the paper allows. Unfold the half moon of paper into a circle. Brush one half with olive oil, and divide the quinoa, vegetables, and fish pieces (skin-side down) between the four oiled halves. Top each piece of cod with 3 to 4 blood orange slices. Drizzle a few spoonfuls of marinade over the fish.

6. To seal the packets, fold the top half of parchment over the fish and align the edges. Starting at one corner, fold over about ½-inch of the edge 3 times, pressing down to make a crisp crease after each fold. Continue to work your way around the edge of the packet, making overlapping, pleat-like folds, always pressing firmly and creasing the edge so the folds hold. When you get to the end of the paper, twist it into a tail to prevent the liquid from seeping out. If necessary, make a second fold wherever there doesn't appear to be a tight seal. When finished, your packet will look like a large calzone.

7. Place the packets on a rimmed baking sheet. Bake for 15 minutes. The paper will darken and puff up as the packet fills with steam. Cooking time will depend on

the thickness of your fish; allow a few more minutes if your filets are more than 1-inch thick.

8. To serve, transfer the packets to a plate. Using scissors or a sharp knife, slit open the lids of the packets and fold the paper back. Sprinkle with flaky salt and top with cilantro leaves, if using.

Prep Time: 30 minutes

Cook Time: 45 minutes

Servings: 4

Ingredients

- 1 tsp ground cumin
- 1 tsp ground coriander
- 1/2 tsp cinnamon
- 1/2 tsp red pepper flakes
- 1 tbsp extra virgin olive oil
- 1 yellow onion chopped into 1-inch pieces
- 1/2 tsp coarse salt plus more to taste
- 2 garlic cloves minced
- 1 tsp grated fresh ginger
- 1/2 cup preserved lemon rinsed and cut into slivers
- 1/2 cups vegetable broth
- 8 dried figs diced
- 2 medium sweet potatoes cut into 1-inch pieces
- 4 medium carrots purple and red, cut into 1-inch pieces

- 3 small green zucchini cut into 1-inch pieces
- 1/2 cups cooked chickpeas drained and rinsed
- 2 tbsp fresh lemon juice
- freshly ground black pepper
- 1/2 cup fresh mint choppped
- 1/4 cup sliced almonds toasted
- Homemade Harissa for serving

Instructions

1. In a small bowl, mix together the cumin, coriander, cinnamon, and red pepper flakes. Set aside.

2. Heat the olive oil in a large pot or Dutch oven over medium heat. Add the onion and the salt and cook until soft, about 5 minutes.

3. Reduce the heat to low and stir in the garlic, ginger, preserved lemon, and dried spices. Add the broth, figs, vegetables, and chickpeas. Bring to a gentle boil, then reduce the heat to low and simmer and cook, covered, for 20 minutes.

4. Cook uncovered for about 8 to 10 minutes, stirring occasionally. Once the stew has thickened and the vegetables are al dente, remove from the heat. Add lemon juice and season with salt and freshly ground pepper.

5. Top with mint and almonds just before serving. Serve with Cauliflower Couscous and Homemade Harissa.

Prep Time: 45 minutes

Cook Time: 20 minutes

Servings: 6

Ingredients

- 1 cup cooked quinoa
- 1 15-ounce can chickpeas liquid included
- 2/3 cup grated carrot
- 2 cloves garlic mashed
- 1 Tablespoon ground cumin
- 1/2 teaspoon smoked paprika
- 1/4 cup chopped fresh parsley
- 1/2 teaspoon salt
- 1 egg beaten
- 1/3 cup whole wheat bread crumbs
- 1/4 cup chickpea flour or all purpose flour
- 1/4 cup extra virgin olive oil for cooking
- 2 avocados skin removed and pit taken out, thinly sliced
- 4 Roma tomatoes thinly sliced

- 10 whole wheat mini buns optional

Instructions

1. In a large bowl combine quinoa and chickpeas. Using a potato masher, break up chickpeas until mostly mashed, a little chunky is ok. Add carrot, garlic, cumin, paprika, parsley, salt, pepper, egg, breadcrumbs and flour. Mix until combined. Add a little water if dry. Should be slightly sticky.

2. Using a 1/3 measuring cup, scoop out mixture and form into patties. Place on a plate and refrigerate covered for up to 2 hours or put in the freezer for 30 minutes. The colder the patties, the better the shape will hold when cooking.

3. Bring a large pan to medium high heat. Add enough oil to thinly coat the bottom of the pan, heat for 60 seconds. Carefully add patties one at a time. Cook 3-5 minutes per side or until a light golden crust appears. Add more oil if pan gets dry.

4. To serve: Place patties on bun. Top with 1-2 slices of avocado and 2 slices of tomato.

Prep Time: 15-20 mins

Cook Time: 15-20 mins

Total Time: 30-40 mins

Yield: Makes 12 mini cakes

Ingredients

Bundt Cakes:

- ¼ cup melted butter
- ¼ cup oil
- ¼ cup dark brown sugar
- 4 large eggs
- 1 teaspoon pure vanilla extract
- 2 cups old-fashioned rolled oats
- 1 cup whole wheat pastry flour
- 2 tablespoons ground flax seed
- ½ teaspoon baking soda
- ¼ teaspoon coarse salt
- ⅔ cup vanilla or plain Greek yogurt
- ⅓ cup milk

Peaches:

- 3 tablespoons melted butter
- 3 tablespoons dark brown sugar
- 2 medium peaches, thinly sliced

Instructions

1. Preheat oven to 350 degrees.

2. In the bowl of a stand mixer, whisk together melted butter, oil and brown sugar until fluffy. Add eggs, one at a time, then vanilla extract and mix until incorporated.

3. In a separate mixing bowl, whisk together oats, flour, flax seed, baking soda and salt. In a measuring cup, whisk together yogurt and milk.

4. Turn the stand mixer on low and add a third of the dry mixture, then half of the yogurt/milk, then repeat, finishing with the dry mixture, just until incorporated.

5. Coat a 12-cup mini bundt pan with cooking spray.

6. In a bowl, stir together melted butter, brown sugar and peach slices. Layer 3 peach slices in the bottom of each well, then fill ¾ of the way full with cake batter. Set aside remaining butter/brown sugar mixture.

7. Bake mini cakes for 15 minutes, or until a toothpick inserted into the center comes out clean. Allow to cool, then remove cakes from the pan. Microwave butter/brown sugar mixture for 30 seconds, or until melted. Pour over each mini bundt cake and top with chopped walnuts (if desired). Serve.

17. Avocado Chocolate Donuts

Prep Time: 10-15 mins

Cook Time: 10-15 mins

Total Time: 20-30 mins

Yield: Makes 12 donuts

Ingredients

Donuts:

- 1 ½ cups oat or whole wheat flour*
- 3 tablespoons dark cocoa powder
- 1 teaspoon baking powder
- 1 teaspoon baking soda
- ⅛ teaspoon coarse salt
- 1 medium ripe avocado, mashed (about ½ cup)
- 1 large egg
- ½ cup granulated sugar
- 2 tablespoons olive oil
- 1 cup milk
- 1 ½ teaspoons pure vanilla extract

Glaze:

- ⅓ cup dark chocolate chips or chunks
- ½ medium ripe avocado, mashed (about ¼ cup)
- 2 tablespoons milk

Toppings:

- 2 tablespoons chopped pistachios or almonds
- 1 tablespoon unsweetened coconut flakes

Instructions

1. Preheat oven to 350 degrees. Coat a donut baking pan with cooking spray. Set aside.
2. Sift oat flour, cocoa powder, baking powder, baking soda and salt into a large mixing bowl.
3. In a separate mixing bowl, use a hand mixer to beat avocado and egg, until smooth. Add sugar and olive oil and beat until smooth. Once fluffy, whisk in milk and vanilla extract until incorporated.
4. Pour wet mixture into dry ingredients while beating on low. Increase the mixed speed to medium and beat until well incorporated. Use a spatula to stir in any

remaining dry mixture on the sides or bottom of the bowl.

5. Pour batter into each well of the prepared donut pan about ¾ of the way to the top (about ¼ cup in each), but not covering the donut hole center. Bake for 13-15 minutes, until toothpick inserted into the center comes out clean. Remove from oven and allow to slightly cool. Flip them onto a baking sheet fitted with a wire rack.

6. In a small bowl, microwave dark cacao for 30 seconds on high. Stir until fully melted. Use hand mixer to beat in avocado on high until very smooth, then beat in milk. Pour a tablespoon of glaze onto each donut. Top with nuts and/or coconut and serve.

18. Carrot Cake Cookie Sandwiches

Prep Time: 15-20 mins

Cook Time: 8-10 mins

Total Time: 23-30 mins

Yield: Makes 8 sandwiches

Ingredients

Carrot Cake Cookies:

- 1 ¾ cups whole wheat flour*
- 1 ½ teaspoons baking powder
- 1 ½ teaspoons ground cinnamon
- ¼ teaspoon ground cloves
- ¼ teaspoon ground nutmeg
- Pinch coarse salt
- ½ cup brown sugar or honey
- ¼ cup soft butter or oil
- 2 large eggs
- 1 teaspoon pure vanilla extract
- 1 cup grated carrots
- ¼ cup golden raisins

Cream Cheese Filling:

- 4-ounces Neufchatel cheese or mascarpone
- 2 ½ tablespoons powdered sugar
- ¼ teaspoon pure vanilla extract
- 2 tablespoons unsweetened coconut flakes (optional)

Instructions

1. In a medium mixing bowl, whisk together flour, baking powder, cinnamon, cloves, nutmeg and salt. Set aside.

2. In another medium mixing bowl, use a hand mixer on medium speed to whip together brown sugar/honey and butter/oil. Once fluffy, add eggs, one at a time until incorporated. Whisk in vanilla extract.

3. Slowing whisk wet ingredient mixture into dry ingredients, on low, until incorporated. Fold in carrots and raisins. Place batter in the refrigerator for 30 minutes.

4. Preheat oven to 325 degrees. Use a medium cookie scoop to form 2-inch mounds on a baking sheet lined

with parchment paper, about 2 inches apart. Bake 8-10 minutes, until soft but slightly browned. Allow to completely cool.

5. To make filling, whip cream cheese/mascarpone on high with a hand mixer or in a stand mixer until fluffy. Whip in sugar and vanilla extract.

6. Spread a 1-inch layer of filling onto the bottom side of half of the cookies. Place remaining cookies on top of the filling, bottom side down, to form cookie sandwiches. Roll edges in coconut, if desired. Keep refrigerated.

19. Apple Fritter Mascarpone Shortcake Bars

Prep Time: 15 mins

Cook Time: 45 mins

Total Time: 60 mins

Yield: 16 bars

Ingredients

Shortcake

- 8 tablespoons butter, softened
- ⅓ cup brown sugar
- 1 cup flour (any variety)
- 1 tablespoon corn starch
- ¼ teaspoon coarse salt
- Mascarpone Filling
- 1 (8 oz.) tub mascarpone
- 2 tablespoons honey
- 1 large egg
- 1 ½ teaspoons vanilla extract
- Apple Fritter
- 1 large or 2 small apples (any variety), sliced

- ¼ cup rolled old-fashioned oats
- 1 ½ tablespoons honey
- 1 ½ teaspoons ground cinnamon

Instructions

1. Preheat oven to 325 degrees.

2. In a mixing bowl, cream butter and brown sugar with a hand mixer, until fluffy. Slowly mix in flour, corn starch and salt, until mixture forms small pea-sized balls (like pie dough). Press into an ungreased 8- or 9-inch brownie pie. Bake 10 minutes, until shortcake starts to rise. Remove from oven and allow to slightly cool.

3. In a separate mixing bowl, whip mascarpone, honey, egg and vanilla extract with a hand mixer, until fluffy. When shortcake is slightly cooled, pour mixture onto the crust and spread evenly.

4. In a mixing bowl, toss apple slices, oats, honey and cinnamon until combined. Line apple slices on mascarpone filling, and sprinkle with remaining oat topping. Bake 35-40 minutes, until mascarpone filling

is set. Allow to completely cool in the refrigerator or freezer before slicing.

20. Cranberry and Goat Cheese Stuffed Pears

Prep Time: 15-20 mins

Cook Time: 20-25 mins

Total Time: 35-45 mins

Yield: Serves 8

Ingredients

- 1 ½ cups fresh cranberries
- 7 tablespooons honey, divided
- 4 medium red or green Bartlett pears
- 2 tablespoons fresh lemon juice
- 4-ounces goat cheese
- ¼ cup old-fashioned rolled oats
- 2 tablespoons chopped walnuts or pecans
- Pinch ground cinnamon + more for topping
- 2 teaspoons butter, melted
- 2 teaspoons brown sugar

Instructions

1. Preheat oven to 425 degrees.

2. In a small saucepan, heat cranberries, ¼ cup water
    and 5 tablespoons honey to medium-high heat. Bring
    to a simmer and allow to cook about 4-5 minutes,
    until cranberries just start to soften and mixture has
    slightly thickened. Remove from heat.

3. Trim a small slice off each side of the pears. Cut in
    half lengthwise. Hollow just the center of the pears
    with a melon baller or spoon, creating a cavity for
    filling. Rub each pear with lemon juice. Bake 17-20
    minutes, until just tender (if pear is ripe, it will take
    less time to cook).

4. In a small bowl, beat goat cheese and remaining 2
    tablespoons honey with a hand mixer until smooth
    and creamy. Place a spoonful of goat cheese mixture
    into each pear. Place a spoonful of cranberry mixture
    into each pear, next to the goat cheese mixture.

5. In another small bowl, mix together oats, walnuts, cinnamon, melted butter and brown sugar. Place a spoonful of oat mixture on each pear.

6. Serve with a sprinkle of cinnamon.

DINNERS

21. Peanut Chicken Curry

Prep Time: 15 min

Cook Time: 20 min

Total Time: 35 min

Yield: Serves 8

Ingredients

- 2 tablespoons oil
- 1 medium yellow onion, peeled and diced
- 2 pounds boneless skinless chicken thighs, diced
- 3 cups fresh spinach
- 3–4 cloves garlic, peeled and minced
- 2-inch piece fresh ginger, peeled and minced
- 2 tablespoons garam masala
- ½ tablespoon ground turmeric
- 2 teaspoons kosher or sea salt
- ½ teaspoon ground black pepper
- ¼ teaspoon ground cayenne pepper
- 2 (15-ounce) cans chickpeas, rinsed and drained

- 1 (15-ounce) can petite diced tomatoes, drained
- 1 (8.25-ounce) container Kitchen Basics Original Chicken Bone Broth (or 1 cup)
- ¾ cup canned coconut milk (the solid top only)
- ¼ cup peanut butter
- 1 ½ tablespoons honey
- Zest and juice of 1 medium lime
- ½ cup fresh cilantro leaves, chopped, divided
- ½ cup roasted peanuts, crushed

Instructions

Stove-Top Directions:

1. Heat oil in a Dutch oven or pot to medium heat. Add onion and saute 2-3 minutes, then add chicken and saute 6-7 minutes or until chicken is browned on the edges, stirring occasionally. Add the spinach, garlic and ginger and saute another 2-3 minutes or until spinach is wilted. Stir in garam masala, turmeric, salt, black pepper and cayenne pepper.

2. Add chickpeas, tomatoes, bone broth (or stock), coconut milk and peanut butter. Let simmer 10-15 minutes.

3. Stir in honey, lime and ¼ cup chopped cilantro. Taste and adjust seasoning, if necessary.

4. Serve over cooked brown or Jasmine rice and top with crushed peanuts.

Pressure Cooker Directions:

1. Place all ingredients, except honey, lime juice, cilantro and peanuts, into the pressure cooker. Stir to combine. Set on high pressure, sealed, for 11 minutes.

2. Once the 11-minute timer goes off, let sit 5 minutes. Carefully use a wooden spoon to flip from sealed to venting and let the steam escape. Once finished, carefully open the lid.

3. Stir in honey, lime and ¼ cup chopped cilantro. Taste and adjust seasoning, if necessary.

4. Serve over cooked brown or Jasmine rice and top with crushed peanuts.

Slow Cooker Directions:

1. Place all ingredients, except honey, lime juice, cilantro and peanuts into the bowl of a slow cooker. Stir to combine. Cook on low 6-8 hours or high 2-3 hours.

2. Stir in honey, lime and ¼ cup chopped cilantro. Taste and adjust seasoning, if necessary.

3. Serve over cooked brown or Jasmine rice and top with crushed peanuts.

22. Butternut Squash Mac & Cheese

Prep Time: 20 min

Cook Time: 1 hr

Total Time: 1 hr 20 min

Yield: Serves 8

Ingredients

- 1 large butternut squash, about 3 pounds*
- ¼ cup water
- 1-pound cavatappi, uncooked
- 3 tablespoons plain Greek yogurt
- 1 ½ cups nonfat milk
- 1 ¼ cups low sodium vegetable or chicken broth
- 1 ½–2 teaspoons coarse salt
- ½ teaspoon ground black pepper
- ¼ teaspoon each nutmeg and cayenne pepper
- 3 tablespoons salted butter
- 2 ½ cups shredded marble jack cheese
- ½ cup shredded Gruyere cheese
- ½ cup shredded Parmesan cheese, divided
- ½ cup panko breadcrumbs

- ¼ cup chopped fresh parsley

Instructions

1. Preheat oven to 375 degrees. Cut butternut squash in half, lengthwise, and scoop out seeds. Place in baking dish, flesh side down, and pour water in the baking dish. Roast in oven for 35-40 minutes, until soft. Scoop out cooked flesh and discard skin. Set squash flesh aside.

2. Cook pasta according to package directions, omitting salt. Drain and set aside.

3. Meanwhile, place butternut squash, Greek yogurt, milk, chicken broth, salt, black pepper, nutmeg and cayenne in a blender and puree until smooth. (If squash is still hot, remove plastic cap from blender lid and place a kitchen towel over it so steam can escape and the hot contents don't explode.)

4. Heat butter in a saucepan and add squash puree. Add marble jack, Gruyere and half of the Parmesan cheese

and cook on medium, stirring, until cheese is melted. Taste and adjust seasoning, if necessary.

5. Coat a 13×9 baking dish with cooking spray. Add cooked pasta to the baking dish and pour in the squash/cheese sauce. Stir until combined. Place in oven and bake for 20 minutes.

6. Remove dish and turn oven on low broil. Top pasta with remaining Parmesan cheese and bread crumbs. Spray top with cooking spray. Place back in the oven and broil for 4-5 minutes, until top is browned, rotating the dish if necessary.

7. Remove from the oven and sprinkle with parsley.

23. Swedish Meatballs

Prep Time: 20 min

Cook Time: 25 min

Total Time: 45 min

Yield: Serves 8

Ingredients

Noodles:

- 12-ounces egg noodles

Meatballs:

- 1-pound ground beef
- 1-pound ground pork
- 2 large eggs
- ½ cup panko breadcrumbs
- 2 tablespoons Dijon mustard
- 1 tablespoon minced onion
- 1 tablespoon Italian seasoning
- 1 ½ teaspoon garlic powder
- 1 ½ teaspoon coarse salt

- ¾ teaspoon ground black pepper
- 2 tablespoons olive oil

Sauce:

- 2 tablespoons butter
- ¼ cup all-purpose flour
- 2 cups unsalted beef stock
- ¾ cup milk
- 1 tablespoon Worcestershire sauce
- ½ tablespoon Dijon mustard
- 1 teaspoon coarse salt
- ½ teaspoon ground black pepper
- ¼ teaspoon ground nutmeg
- ¼ teaspoon cayenne pepper
- ¼ cup flat-leaf Italian parsley, chopped (optional)

Instructions

1. Bring a large pot of salted water to a boil. Cook egg noodles according to package directions. Drain and set aside.

2. In a medium bowl, combine meatball ingredients, except the olive oil. Roll mixture into 2-inch meatballs.

3. Heat olive oil in a Dutch oven to medium heat. Sauté meatballs in the oil 8-10 minutes or until meatballs are firm, turning occasionally so each side browns. Transfer to a plate.

4. Add butter to the Dutch oven and whisk in flour until it's bubbly and lightly browned. Slowly whisk in beef stock, then milk. Stir in Worcestershire sauce, Dijon, salt, black pepper, nutmeg and cayenne. Bring to a simmer for 4-5 minutes or until thickened, whisking frequently. Taste and adjust seasoning, if necessary. Add meatballs over egg noodles. Garnish with parsley, if desired.

24. Spaghetti Squash with Italian Meatballs & Creamy Tomato Sauce

Prep Time: 20 min

Cook Time: 45 min

Total Time: 1 hr 5 min

Yield: Serves 8

Ingredients

Spaghetti Squash:

- 2 medium spaghetti squashes

Creamy Tomato Sauce:

- 1 tablespoon olive oil
- ½ medium yellow or white onion, peeled and diced
- 2–3 cloves garlic, peeled and minced
- 1 tablespoon Italian seasoning
- ½ tablespoon dried oregano leaves
- 1 (32-ounce) can whole San Marzano tomatoes
- ¼ cup fresh basil leaves
- 1 teaspoon coarse salt

- ½ teaspoon freshly ground black pepper
- ¼ teaspoon crushed red pepper flakes
- 1 ½ teaspoons granulated sugar
- 2-ounces (about ¼ cup) cream cheese

Italian Meatballs:

- ½-pound lean ground beef
- ½-pound ground Italian sausage or ground pork
- 2 large eggs
- ½ cup Panko breadcrumbs
- 2 tablespoons freshly grated Parmesan
- 1 tablespoon Dijon mustard
- ½ tablespoon dried oregano leaves
- ½ teaspoon coarse salt
- ¼ teaspoon ground black pepper

Garnishes:

- ¼ cup freshly grated Parmesan cheese
- ¼ cup flat-leaf Italian parsley, chopped

Instructions

1. To make spaghetti squash: Slice spaghetti squashes in half and scoop out the seeds. Place face-down in a baking dish. Pour ½ cup water into the dish. Microwave on high 10-12 minutes, or until fork-tender or bake at 400 degrees for 45-60 minutes, or until fork-tender. Let slightly cool, then use a fork to loosen strands of squash. For serving, leave squash strands in the shell or remove and place in bowls.

2. To make tomato sauce: Heat oil in a Dutch oven or high-sided pan to medium-low heat. Add onion and sauté 6-7 minutes or until soft. Stir in garlic, Italian seasoning and oregano. Add tomatoes and fresh basil and bring to a simmer. Crush the tomatoes with a wooden spoon, then let simmer 10-15 minutes. Stir in salt and black pepper. Use an immersion blender to puree the sauce until very smooth, or transfer mixture to a blender and puree until very smooth. Stir in sugar and cream cheese until cream cheese is melted. Taste and adjust seasoning, if necessary.

3. To make meatballs: Preheat oven to 375 degrees. Fit a baking sheet with a wire rack and coat with cooking

spray. Place all ingredients into a large bowl and mix with your hands until ingredients are thoroughly combined. Form into 2-inch meatballs and place on the prepared rack. Bake 17-20 minutes or until meatballs are set and internal temperature reaches 155 degrees.

4. Serve spaghetti squash with meatballs and creamy tomato sauce, and garnish with chopped parsley and Parmesan cheese.

25. Rustic Heirloom Tomato Pizza

Prep Time: 15 min

Cook Time: 25 min

Total Time: 40 min

Yield: 1 pizza / Serves 4

Ingredients

Pizza Crust:

- 1 ¾ cups whole wheat pastry flour
- 1 teaspoon baking powder
- ½ teaspoon coarse salt
- 1 ½ cups plain Greek yogurt
- 1–2 tablespoons olive oil

Pizza:

- 4-ounces boursin cheese (with herbs)
- 3–4 medium heirloom tomatoes, sliced
- Coarse salt and freshly cracked black pepper
- 4–5 sprigs fresh thyme, stems removed

Instructions

1. Preheat oven to 425 degrees.

2. In a large bowl, mix together flour, baking powder, salt and Greek yogurt until a dough ball forms. Transfer to a baking sheet or pizza stone and press into a ¼-inch thick round and brush olive oil over the top. Bake 5-7 minutes. Remove from the oven.

3. Drop clumps of boursin cheese on the crust, then top with slices of tomato and sprinkle with salt and freshly ground black pepper. Bake an additional 10-12 minutes, then turn the oven to a low broil. Broil 3-4 minutes or until cheese is browned and bubbly.

4. Let slightly cool, then slice into wedges and top with fresh thyme leaves.

26. Restaurant-Style Beef and Broccoli Stir Fry

Prep Time: 15 min

Cook Time: 25 min

Total Time: 40 min

Yield: Serves 4

Ingredients

- 1 egg white
- 1 tablespoon rice wine (or mirin)
- 2 tablespoons cornstarch, divided
- ¼ teaspoon coarse salt
- 1-pound beef top loin or flank steak, thinly sliced against the grain
- ¼ cup unsalted beef stock
- 3 tablespoons oyster sauce
- 2 tablespoons rice wine (or mirin)
- 2 tablespoons low sodium soy sauce
- 1 tablespoon brown sugar
- 2 teaspoons sesame oil
- 3 tablespoons oil
- 1 medium head broccoli, cut into florets (about 3–4 cups)

- 2-inch piece ginger, peeled and minced
- 2–3 cloves garlic, peeled and minced
- Cooked rice, sesame seeds and sliced green onion, for serving

Instructions

1. In a medium glass mixing bowl, whisk together egg white, rice wine, 1 tablespoon cornstarch and salt until thoroughly combined. Add strips of beef and toss to combine. Marinate for about 30 minutes in the refrigerator.

2. In a separate bowl, whisk together beef stock, oyster sauce, rice wine, soy sauce, brown sugar and sesame oil. Vigorously whisk in remaining 1 tablespoon cornstarch until smooth. Set aside.

3. Heat oil to medium-high in a large skillet or wok. In batches, sauté marinated beef strips for 1-2 minutes, flipping once, until browned and crispy on all edges. Remove cooked beef and place on a paper towel-lined plate. Add broccoli florets to the hot skillet or wok and sauté 3-4 minutes, until just tender, stirring frequently. Stir in ginger and garlic and sauté an additional 30-60 seconds.

4. Pour sauce into the wok or skillet and simmer 1-2 minutes, until thickened.

5. Serve beef & broccoli over cooked rice and top with sesame seeds and green onion.

27. Moroccan Lamb Lollipops

Prep Time: 5 min

Cook Time: 10 min

Total Time: 15 min

Yield: Serves 8

Ingredients

- 2 tablespoons ground cumin
- 1 ½ tablespoons ground coriander
- 1 tablespoon paprika or smoked paprika
- 2 teaspoons each ground turmeric, ground ginger and ground cinnamon
- 1 teaspoon each coarse salt and ground black pepper
- ½ teaspoon allspice and cayenne pepper
- Pinch ground cloves
- 2 pounds rack of lamb, cut into lollipops
- 1–2 tablespoons olive oil

Instructions

1. In a small bowl, whisk together cumin, coriander, paprika, turmeric, ginger, cinnamon, salt, pepper, allspice, cayenne and cloves until combined.

2. Place lamb lollipops on a baking sheet and evenly coat with spice rub on all sides.

3. Heat oil in a large cast iron skillet to medium or medium-high heat.

   Work in batches to pan-fry lamb lollipops, about 2-3 minutes per side, just until browned and crispy on both sides. Lollipops are best cooked medium-rare to medium (140-145 degrees).

Prep Time: 15 minutes

Cook Time: 10 minutes

Total Time: 25 minutes

Yield: Serves 8

Ingredients

- 1-pound tagliatelle
- 1 cup pitted Mediterranean olives
- 1 cup flat-leaf Italian parsley
- ¼ cup pine nuts or walnuts
- 1 teaspoon dried oregano leaves
- ¼ teaspoon freshly cracked black pepper + more for serving
- 1–2 cloves garlic, peeled
- ¼ cup + 2 tablespoons olive oil + more for serving
- 8-ounces fresh mini mozzarella balls

Instructions

1. Bring a large pot of salted water to a boil. Cook tagliatelle according to package directions. Drain.

2. Place olives, parsley, nuts, oregano, black pepper, garlic and olive oil in the bowl of a food processor. Pulse until desired consistency is reached, scraping the sides of the bowl as needed.

3. Toss olive pesto with hot pasta, adding olive oil as desired.

4. Serve in bowls with mini mozzarella balls and freshly cracked black pepper.

Prep Time: 30 mins

Cook Time: 20 mins

Total Time: 50 mins

Yield: 8 Servings

Ingredients

- ¼ cup butter or olive oil
- 2 tablespoons non-pareil capers, drained
- 1 cup (8-ounces) ricotta (whole milk or part skim)
- ⅓ cup shredded mozzarella
- 2 cups baby spinach, finely chopped
- ¾ cup (~7.5-ounce jar) quartered marinated artichoke hearts, drained and roughly chopped
- 2 cloves garlic, peeled and minced
- ½ teaspoon freshly ground black pepper, divided
- ¼ teaspoon kosher salt
- Pinch crushed red pepper flakes
- 48 wonton wrappers
- ½ cup freshly shaved Parmesan

Instructions

1. Bring a gallon of salted water to a boil.

2. Melt butter on low heat in a small saucepan (or heat olive oil to warm temperature). Stir in capers. Shut off the heat and leave saucepan on the burner while preparing ravioli.

3. To a medium mixing bowl, add ricotta, mozzarella, chopped baby spinach, artichoke hearts, garlic, ¼ teaspoon black pepper, salt and crushed red pepper flakes. Mix to thoroughly combine.

4. Line 24 wonton wrappers on a cutting board. Spoon a rounded tablespoon of filling in the center of each wrapper. Lightly brush edge of each wrapper with water, then place a second wrapper on top and seal, pressing out trapped air. Repeat with remaining wrappers and filling. Press the edges of each ravioli with a fork to create decorative edges.

5. Boil ravioli in 3-4 batches until tender, 2 to 3 minutes per batch, removing with a slotted spoon and placing in six serving bowls.

6. Spoon caper butter over ravioli and garnish with shaved Parmesan and remaining ¼ teaspoon black pepper.

30. Asian Pork Meatballs with Sesame Cucumber Salad

Prep Time: 15 mins

Cook Time: 20 mins

Total Time: 35 mins

Yield: Serves 4

Ingredients

Pork Meatballs

- 1 pound ground pork
- 2 large eggs
- 1 cup Panko breadcrumbs
- ¼ cup cilantro leaves, chopped
- 2 tablespoons brown sugar
- 1 tablespoon soy sauce
- 2 teaspoon Sriracha or gochujang
- 2 cloves garlic, minced
- 1-inch piece fresh ginger, peeled and minced
- ¾ teaspoon coarse salt
- ½ teaspoon ground black pepper

Cucumber Salad:

- 1 large English cucumber, shaved
- 1 large carrot, peeled and shaved
- 1 tablespoon rice wine vinegar
- 1 teaspoon sesame oil
- Pinch coarse salt and crushed red pepper flakes

Instructions

1. Preheat oven to 375 degrees. Coat a baking sheet fitted with a wire rack with cooking spray. Set aside.

2. To make meatballs, thoroughly mix all of the meatball ingredients together in a bowl. Form 2-inch meatballs and place on the wire rack about an inch apart. Bake 15-18 minutes, until internal temperature of meatballs reaches 145 degrees.

3. To make cucumber salad, toss together all ingredients. Taste and adjust seasoning, if necessary.

4. Serve salad with meatballs.